Gastritis-Friendly smoothies:

Delicious and nourishing blends for a healthy digestive system

By Donna Nettles

TABLE OF CONTENTS

INTRODUCTION

CHAPTER 1: What is Gastritis

CHAPTER 2: Benefits Of Smoothies For Gastritis

CHAPTER 3: Nutritional Considerations For Gastritis Sufferers

CHAPTER 4: Delicious Recipes for Gastritis-Friendly Smoothies

CHAPTER 5: Tips for Making the Perfect Gastritis-Friendly Smoothie

CONCLUSION

INTRODUCTION

Nora was a 40-year-old woman who was suffering from severe gastritis. She had been suffering from the condition for years and had tried various medications and treatments but none of them seemed to be helping her. She had lost hope and was resigned to living with the condition for the rest of her life.

One day, she came across an article about how smoothies could be beneficial for people with gastritis. She decided to give it a try and started making her smoothies. She began with simple ingredients like fresh fruits and vegetables, yogurt, nuts, and honey. She discovered that the smoothies were not only delicious but also very beneficial for her gastritis.

With time, Nora tweaked her smoothie recipes and started adding more ingredients like herbs, spices, and probiotics. She found out that these ingredients not only made her smoothies more flavorful but also helped in reducing her gastritis symptoms. She also started drinking her smoothies regularly and soon, she was feeling much better.

Her gastritis symptoms had improved significantly and she was able to live a much more comfortable life without any pain or discomfort. She was amazed by the results and began recommending her smoothie recipes to her friends and family, who also found relief from their gastritis symptoms.

Nora continued to experiment with her smoothie recipes and eventually came up with a recipe that was perfect for her condition. She was now able to enjoy her life without any gastritis symptoms and was proud of the fact that she had been able to heal herself with just smoothies.

Nora's success story is an inspiration for anyone suffering from gastritis and it shows us that there is hope for those who are suffering from this condition. We may not be able to control our bodies but we can certainly control what we put into them, and Nora's story proves that with the right ingredients and a healthy lifestyle, we can heal ourselves.

Understanding gastric health

Gastric health is an essential component of overall health and well-being. It is essential for the proper functioning of the digestive system and the absorption of nutrients from food. Gastric health is affected by a variety of factors, including diet, lifestyle, and medical conditions. Understanding the factors that affect gastric health and how to maintain it is an important part of managing overall health.

Gastric health is vital for the proper digestion and absorption of food. Gastric health includes the production of digestive enzymes, the breakdown of food components, and the absorption of nutrients. The stomach is the first step in the digestion process, and various factors can impact how it functions. These include diet, lifestyle, and medical conditions.

Diet is an important factor in maintaining gastric health. Eating a balanced diet and avoiding foods that are high in sugar, fat, and processed ingredients can help to promote healthy digestion. Eating several small meals throughout the day, instead of two or three large meals, can also help to maintain healthy gastric function.

Lifestyle factors can also have an impact on gastric health. Stress can trigger an increase in stomach acid, which can lead to indigestion and other digestive issues. Getting plenty of rest, exercising regularly, and practicing relaxation techniques can help to reduce stress and improve overall health.

Certain medical conditions can also affect gastric health. Gastroesophageal reflux disease (GERD) is a common condition that causes acid reflux and other digestive problems. Other medical conditions, such as Crohn's disease and ulcerative colitis, can also affect gastric health.

In addition to diet and lifestyle, various supplements and medications can help to promote gastric health. Probiotics, which are beneficial bacteria that help to support healthy digestion, are available in supplement form. Antacids, which neutralize stomach acid to relieve indigestion, can also be helpful. It is important to talk to a doctor before taking any supplements or medications for gastric health.

Understanding the factors that affect gastric health and how to maintain it is an essential part of managing overall health. Eating a balanced diet, getting plenty of rest, and reducing stress can help to promote healthy digestion. Certain supplements and medications can also be used to support gastric health. In addition, it is important to talk to a doctor if symptoms of digestive issues persist.

Smoothies are a great way to get the essential vitamins and minerals needed to help fight off gastritis. They are also incredibly easy to make, and they can be tailored to your specific needs.

In this book, I will discuss the various types of smoothies that can help alleviate the symptoms of gastritis, as well as provide delicious recipes to help make the process of creating smoothies much easier. I will also offer some tips and tricks for making sure your smoothies are as nutritious and beneficial as possible. So, if you are looking for a way to reduce the symptoms of gastritis and improve your overall health, then this book is for you!

CHAPTER 1: What is Gastritis

Gastritis is a medical condition that affects the lining of the stomach. The condition is characterized by inflammation of the stomach lining, which can cause pain, nausea, vomiting, bloating, and other symptoms. The stomach lining, or mucosa, is composed of several layers of cells. These cells help to protect the stomach from the acidic digestive juices produced by the stomach. When these cells become damaged, the stomach becomes vulnerable to irritation and inflammation. This is what is known as gastritis. Acute or chronic gastritis is also possible.

Acute Gastritis

Acute gastritis is a sudden inflammation that can last from a few hours to a few days. Acute gastritis is a condition in which the stomach lining becomes inflamed, irritated, and swollen. It is usually caused by infection, excessive alcohol consumption, or the regular use of certain medications. In some cases, acute gastritis can also be caused by an autoimmune reaction, in which the body's immune system mistakenly attacks the stomach lining.

The most common symptoms of acute gastritis include abdominal pain and discomfort, indigestion, nausea, vomiting, and loss of appetite. Other symptoms may include bloating, belching, and hiccups. In some cases, acute gastritis may cause bleeding in the stomach and a feeling of fullness even after eating only a small amount.

The diagnosis of acute gastritis is usually based on the patient's medical history and a physical examination. Tests such as blood tests, endoscopy, and biopsy may also be used to help diagnose the condition. Treatment of acute gastritis depends on its cause and may include antibiotics, antacids, acid-suppressing medication, or other medications that reduce inflammation.

In most cases, acute gastritis can be successfully managed with proper treatment. However, if left untreated, it can lead to complications such as bleeding, ulcers, perforations, and anemia. Therefore, it is important to seek medical advice if you experience any of the symptoms of acute gastritis.

The most important thing you can do to manage your acute gastritis is to identify and address the underlying cause. If the cause is a bacterial infection, your doctor may prescribe antibiotics to treat it. If the cause is the overuse of certain medications, your doctor may recommend that you stop taking them. If the cause is an autoimmune disease, your doctor may prescribe medications to suppress your immune system.

In addition to treating the underlying cause, your doctor may prescribe medications to reduce your symptoms. Antacids, proton pump inhibitors, and histamine-2 receptor antagonists are a few examples. Also, your doctor could advise that you alter your diet. These may include avoiding foods that are high in fat, avoiding alcohol, and eating smaller meals more frequently.

Chronic Gastritis

Chronic gastritis is a long-term condition that can last for months or even years.

Chronic gastritis is a condition characterized by inflammation of the stomach lining, which can lead to pain, indigestion, and other digestive issues. It is usually caused by an infection with the bacteria Helicobacter pylori (H. pylori) or the regular use of certain medications such as non-steroidal anti-inflammatory drugs (NSAIDs).

Common symptoms of chronic gastritis include abdominal pain, nausea and vomiting, bloating, loss of appetite, and heartburn. In some cases, chronic gastritis may also lead to weight loss, fatigue, and blood in the stool.

Chronic gastritis can be diagnosed by conducting a physical examination and performing a series of tests. These tests may include a complete blood count (CBC), X-rays, a stool sample, an endoscopy, or a biopsy.

The treatment for chronic gastritis typically depends on the cause. If the cause is an infection with H. pylori, the doctor may prescribe antibiotics. If the cause is the regular use of certain medications, the doctor may recommend avoiding or reducing the dose of the medication. In some cases, surgery may be necessary to remove a growth or an ulcer.

The best way to prevent chronic gastritis is to avoid the things that can cause it, such as regular use of certain medications, smoking, and eating a diet high in processed foods. It is also important to practice good hygiene, such as washing your hands before eating, to reduce the risk of infection with H. pylori.

If you have any of the symptoms of chronic gastritis, it is important to see your doctor right away to get a proper diagnosis and treatment.

With the right treatment, chronic gastritis can be managed, and the symptoms will improve.

Generally, there are several causes of gastritis, including bacterial infections, the use of certain medications, alcohol consumption, and autoimmune disorders. Gastritis can be treated with medications, lifestyle changes, and dietary modifications.

The most common symptom of gastritis is a pain in the upper abdomen, usually on the left side. Other symptoms can include nausea and vomiting, bloating, loss of appetite, indigestion, and feeling of fullness after eating. In some cases, it can cause bleeding in the stomach, leading to black or tarry stools.

Gastritis is a very serious condition and can cause complications if left untreated. It can increase the risk of developing various stomach and intestinal conditions, including ulcers, cancer, and perforation of the stomach wall.

Gastritis is often treated with medications that decrease the amount of acid produced by the stomach, as well as antibiotics. These medications help to reduce inflammation and allow the stomach lining to heal. In more severe cases, surgery may be necessary to remove the affected tissue.

Gastritis can be diagnosed through physical examination and various tests, such as endoscopy, biopsy, blood tests, and imaging tests. Treatment usually involves medications, such as proton pump inhibitors and antibiotics, and lifestyle changes, such as avoiding alcohol and smoking. Dietary modifications, such as avoiding certain foods and eating small, frequent meals, can also help reduce symptoms and improve overall health.

When it comes to prevention, the best way to avoid gastritis is to maintain a healthy lifestyle. Eating a balanced diet and avoiding certain foods that are known to trigger gastritis can help. In addition, avoiding smoking and alcohol can help reduce the risk of developing the condition.

It is important to remember that gastritis is a very serious condition that can have serious consequences if it is left untreated. If you experience any of the symptoms of gastritis, it is important to seek medical care right away.

CHAPTER 2: Benefits Of Smoothies For Gastritis

Smoothies are a great way to get some of the essential vitamins and minerals that your body needs, while also being a tasty treat. For those suffering from gastritis, smoothies can provide an easy and delicious way to get the nutrition that your body needs.

While there is no one-size-fits-all diet for gastritis, there are certain foods that can help manage the symptoms. Smoothies can be a great way to get some of these beneficial nutrients without putting too much strain on the digestive system.

Smoothies are easy to make and can be tailored to meet your individual needs. Start with a base of fruit and vegetables for vitamins, minerals, and fiber. Add in a liquid such as almond milk, coconut milk, or even water to thin out the mixture. If you're looking for a protein boost, try adding Greek yogurt, nut butter, or protein powder.

They can also be a great way to incorporate superfoods into your diet. Superfoods are foods that are especially rich in vitamins, minerals, and other nutrients. Examples of superfoods include chia seeds, bee pollen, spirulina, and wheatgrass. These superfoods can help provide extra nutrition to support your body's needs and can be easily blended into your favorite smoothie recipe.

Smoothies are also a great way to get the most out of your food. They are easy to make and can be made in advance for a quick and easy breakfast, snack, or even a meal replacement. When you blend your ingredients, you're able to break down the cells of the food, which makes it easier for your body to absorb the nutrients. This means that you're able to get more out of the foods that you're eating.

They are also a great way to get a lot of nutrients in a single drink as they are packed with fiber, vitamins, minerals, and antioxidants that can help boost your overall health and well-being. Smoothies are also great for maintaining a healthy weight as they can fill you up with fewer calories than a regular meal.

Smoothies are a considerable way to get your day-to-day intake of fruits and vegetables. You can use fresh, frozen, or canned fruit and vegetables to make a delicious and nutritious smoothie. Adding in a few ingredients like nuts and seeds can also give your smoothie an extra boost of protein and healthy fats.

They are also a wonderful way to add variety to your diet. You can mix and match different ingredients to make delicious smoothies with different flavors and textures. You can also get creative and add in ingredients like chia seeds, Greek yogurt, or oats to make a more nutritious smoothie.

Smoothies are also convenient. You can make them ahead of time and store them in the refrigerator for up to a few days. This makes them a great option for busy days when you don't have time to cook.

Overall, smoothies are a great way to get some of the essential vitamins and minerals that your body needs, while also being a delicious treat. With the right ingredients, smoothies can be a great way to manage gastritis symptoms and get the most out of your foods.
Taking smoothies is a great way to get more nutrients into your diet. So, if you want to get more nutrients into your diet, try making a smoothie!

<u>Below are some listed benefits that smoothies can provide, for those with gastritis.</u>

1. High in Nutrients: Smoothies are packed with essential vitamins and minerals, making them a great source of nutrition for people with gastritis.

2. Easy to Digest: The blended nature of smoothies makes them easier to digest than solid foods, which can be difficult for people with gastritis to tolerate.

3. Low Acid: Smoothies are naturally low in acid, which can help reduce inflammation and discomfort associated with gastritis.

4. Antioxidants: Smoothies can be loaded with antioxidants from fresh fruits and vegetables, which can help reduce inflammation and protect the stomach lining from further damage.

5. Immune-Boosting: Many smoothies contain immune-boosting ingredients like berries, greens, and probiotic-rich yogurt, which can help maintain a healthy digestive system and reduce gastritis symptoms.

6. Fiber: Smoothies are a great way to get more fiber into the diet, which can help reduce inflammation and keep the digestive system running smoothly.

7. Hydration: Smoothies are a great way to stay hydrated, which is important for people with gastritis, as dehydration can exacerbate symptoms.

8. Variety: Smoothies offer a lot of variety when it comes to ingredients, which can help keep the diet interesting and make sure you're getting all the nutrients you need.

9. Customization: Smoothies can be customized to meet individual dietary needs and preferences, making them a great choice for people with gastritis.

10. Quick and Convenient: Smoothies are quick and easy to make, making them an ideal choice for busy people with limited time for meal preparation.

11. Delicious: Smoothies are a delicious way to get the nutrients and hydration you need to keep your gastritis under control.

12. Cost-Effective: Smoothies are often cheaper than other meal options, making them a budget-friendly choice for people with gastritis.

13. Versatility: Smoothies can be enjoyed as a snack, a meal replacement, or a post-workout recovery drink, making them a versatile addition to any diet.

14. Stress-Relieving: Drinking a smoothie can be a relaxing and calming experience, which can help reduce stress and its associated symptoms.

15. Easy to Add Supplements: Smoothies are a great way to add supplements to your diet, such as probiotics and digestive enzymes, which can help reduce gastritis symptoms.

16. Low-Calorie: Smoothies are often low in calories, making them a great choice for people looking to lose weight while managing their gastritis.

17. Promote Gut Health: Smoothies can be made with ingredients that support gut health, such as yogurt and other probiotic-rich foods, which can help reduce inflammation and improve overall health.

18. Convenience: Smoothies can be made ahead of time and stored in the fridge or freezer for later, making them a convenient meal option for busy people with gastritis.

19. Comfort: Smoothies can be comforting and soothing, making them a great choice for people with gastritis who need additional relief from their symptoms.

20. Portion Control: Smoothies are a great way to manage portion size, which can be beneficial for people with gastritis who need to watch their intake.

CHAPTER 3: Nutritional Considerations For Gastritis Sufferers

Nutrition plays an important role in the treatment of gastritis, a condition caused by inflammation of the stomach lining. Eating the right foods can help to reduce symptoms and make managing the condition easier.

When it comes to nutrition, gastritis sufferers should focus on eating small, frequent meals throughout the day, with a few snacks in between. This will help to prevent overeating and reduce the risk of irritating the stomach lining. It is important to choose nutrient-dense foods that provide energy and nourishment without taxing the digestive system.

Lean proteins such as fish, chicken, and non-processed red meats are good choices for gastritis sufferers. Plant-based proteins like beans, nuts, and seeds are also beneficial.

Low-fat dairy products and eggs are also great sources of protein, but be sure to avoid any high-fat dairy products.

Fruits and vegetables should be a large part of the diet, as they are rich in vitamins, minerals, and fiber. Focus on eating a variety of fruits and vegetables to get the most nutrients and benefits. Avoid any raw or very acidic fruits and vegetables, as these can aggravate gastritis symptoms.

Whole grains are a great source of fiber and other nutrients and can provide energy and nourishment. Choose whole grains like quinoa, buckwheat, oats, and barley over processed grains like white rice and white bread.

Healthy fats like olive oil, avocado, and nuts are beneficial for gastritis sufferers, as they provide essential fatty acids and help to reduce inflammation. Avoid processed fats like margarine, as they can irritate the stomach lining.

Finally, it is important to stay well-hydrated to help with digestion and prevent dehydration. Avoid sugary and caffeinated drinks, and opt instead for water, herbal teas, or other non-caffeinated beverages.

Gastritis sufferers should also avoid any foods that may worsen symptoms, such as spicy, greasy, and fried foods, as well as processed and packaged foods. Additionally, alcohol should be avoided, as it can irritate the stomach lining.

By following these nutritional guidelines, gastritis sufferers can ensure that their bodies are getting the nourishment they need while reducing the risk of aggravating their symptoms. With proper nutrition and lifestyle changes, managing gastritis can be much easier.

Essential Ingredients for gastritis friendly smoothies

Eating a diet that is both nutritious and gentle on the stomach can help to reduce the symptoms of gastritis and keep the condition under control. Here are some of the *key* ingredients that can help create a gastritis-friendly diet.

1. Fruits and Vegetables: Fruits and vegetables are an essential part of a healthy diet, and they can also be beneficial for people with gastritis. Fruits and vegetables provide vitamins, minerals, and fiber, all of which can help to reduce inflammation and promote healing. Choose fruits and vegetables that are low in acidity, such as apples, bananas, pears, carrots, sweet potatoes, and spinach.

2. Whole Grains: Whole grains such as oats, quinoa, barley, and brown rice provide fiber, vitamins, and minerals, as well as a slow-releasing source of energy that can help to regulate blood sugar levels and reduce inflammation.

3. Lean Protein: Lean protein sources, such as chicken, fish, and legumes, can help to reduce inflammation and provide essential nutrients. Avoid high-fat proteins such as red meat, which can be difficult to digest and can trigger symptoms of gastritis.

4. Healthy Fats: Healthy fats such as avocados, nuts, and seeds are a great source of essential fatty acids, which help to reduce inflammation and improve digestion.

5. Herbs and Spices: Herbs and spices such as turmeric, ginger, and garlic can help to reduce inflammation and provide flavor to dishes without adding salt or sugar.

6. Probiotics: Probiotics are beneficial bacteria that can help to reduce inflammation and improve digestive health. Probiotics can be found in fermented foods such as yogurt, kefir, and sauerkraut, as well as in supplements.

7. Water: Staying hydrated is essential for good health, and it can also help to reduce symptoms of gastritis. Strive for at least 8 glasses of water per day.

These are the essential ingredients for a gastritis-friendly diet. Eating a balanced, nutritious diet and avoiding foods that trigger symptoms can help to reduce the severity of gastritis and keep the condition under control.

<u>Below are examples of some of the essential ingredients, showing their importance to the body</u>

1. Almond Milk: Almond milk is one of the most preferred options for smoothies due to its high calcium, protein, and magnesium content, which are all essential for boosting the digestive system and maintaining overall health.

2. Bananas: Bananas are a great source of dietary fiber and provide a creamy texture to smoothies. They also contain potassium, which is important for maintaining fluid balance and electrolyte levels in the body, preventing dehydration.

3. Avocados: Avocados are high in healthy fats and dietary fiber, which help to improve digestion and reduce inflammation in the stomach. The high levels of potassium in avocados also help to reduce stomach acid.

4. Berries: Berries are a great source of antioxidants, which help to reduce inflammation and protect the body from free radical damage. They are also high in fiber, which helps to improve digestion.

5. Oats: Oats are high in fiber, which helps to reduce inflammation in the stomach and improve digestion. They are also a good source of magnesium, which helps to balance electrolytes in the body.

6. Greek Yogurt: Greek yogurt is high in probiotics, which help to improve digestion and reduce inflammation in the stomach. It's also high in calcium, which helps to reduce stomach acid.

7. Coconut Milk: Coconut milk is a great choice for those with gastritis because it is high in healthy fats, which help to reduce inflammation. The high levels of magnesium in coconut milk also help to reduce stomach acid.

8. Aloe Vera Juice: Aloe vera juice is a great source of antioxidants and helps to reduce inflammation in the stomach. It also helps to improve digestion.

9. Green Tea: Green tea is a great source of antioxidants and helps to reduce inflammation. It also helps to improve digestion.

10. Flaxseed: Flaxseed is high in fiber, which helps to reduce inflammation in the stomach and improve digestion. The omega-3 fatty acids in flaxseed also help to reduce inflammation.

11. Ginger: Ginger is a great source of antioxidants and helps to reduce inflammation in the stomach. It also helps to improve digestion.

12. Turmeric: Turmeric is high in antioxidants and helps to reduce inflammation in the stomach. It also helps to improve digestion.

13. Kefir: Kefir is a fermented milk drink that is high in probiotics, which helps to improve digestion and reduce inflammation in the stomach.

14. Chia Seeds: Chia seeds are a great source of fiber, which helps to reduce inflammation in the stomach and improve digestion. The omega-3 fatty acids in chia seeds also help to reduce inflammation.

15. Spirulina: Spirulina is a type of algae that is high in protein and iron, which helps to reduce inflammation in the stomach. It also helps to improve digestion.

16. Hemp Seeds: Hemp seeds are high in fiber and healthy fats, which help to reduce inflammation in the stomach and improve digestion.

17. Maca Powder: Maca powder is a root vegetable that is high in vitamins and minerals, which helps to reduce inflammation in the stomach. It also helps to improve digestion.

18. Spinach: Spinach is high in fiber and vitamins, which help to reduce inflammation in the stomach and improve digestion.

19. Lettuce: Lettuce is high in fiber and water, which helps to reduce inflammation in the stomach and improve digestion.

20. Cucumber: Cucumber is high in water and dietary fiber, which helps to reduce inflammation in the stomach and improve digestion.

21. Apple Cider Vinegar: Apple cider vinegar is high in acetic acid, which helps to reduce inflammation in the stomach and improve digestion. It also helps to balance stomach acid levels.

22. Lemon Juice: Lemon juice is high in vitamin C, which helps to reduce inflammation in the stomach and improve digestion. It also helps to lower stomach acid.

23. Basil: Basil is high in antioxidants and helps to reduce inflammation in the stomach. It also helps to improve digestion.

24. Parsley: Parsley is high in fiber and vitamins, which help to reduce inflammation in the stomach and improve digestion. It also helps to reduce stomach acid.

25. Cinnamon: Cinnamon is high in antioxidants and helps to reduce inflammation in the stomach. It also helps to improve digestion.

26. Mint: Mint is high in antioxidants and helps to reduce inflammation in the stomach. It also helps to improve digestion.

By including these ingredients in your smoothies, you can create a nutritious and delicious drink that is beneficial for those suffering from gastritis.

CHAPTER 4: Delicious Recipes for Gastritis-Friendly Smoothies

1. Blueberry Banana Smoothie:

Ingredients:

½ cup ripe banana

½ cup blueberries

1 cup non-fat yogurt

½ cup ice cubes

Preparation: Peel and slice the banana, then place it in a blender with the blueberries, yogurt, and ice cubes. Blend until smooth.

Storage: Store in the refrigerator and consume within 24 hours.

2. Avocado Kale Smoothie:

<u>Ingredients:</u>
1 cup kale
½ avocado
½ cup mango
1 cup non-fat yogurt

<u>Preparation:</u> Wash and remove the stems from the kale, then place in a blender with the avocado, mango, and yogurt. Blend until smooth.

<u>Storage:</u> Store in the refrigerator and consume within 24 hours.

3. Pineapple Spinach Smoothie:

<u>Ingredients:</u>
1 cup spinach
½ cup pineapple
1 cup non-fat yogurt
½ cup ice cubes

<u>Preparation:</u> Wash and remove the stems from the spinach, then place in a blender with the

pineapple, yogurt, and ice cubes. Blend until smooth.

Storage: Store in the refrigerator and consume within 24 hours.

4. Mango Coconut Smoothie:
Ingredients:
½ cup mango
½ cup coconut milk
1 teaspoon honey
½ cup ice cubes

Preparation: Peel and slice the mango, then place it in a blender with the coconut milk, honey, and ice cubes. Blend until smooth.

Storage: Store in the refrigerator and consume within 24 hours.

5. Orange Raspberry Smoothie:
Ingredients:
½ cup orange juice
½ cup raspberries

1 cup non-fat yogurt
½ cup ice cubes

Preparation: Place the orange juice, raspberries, yogurt, and ice cubes in a blender. Blend until smooth.

Storage: Store in the refrigerator and consume within 24 hours.

6. Apple Banana Smoothie:
Ingredients:
½ cup ripe banana
½ cup apple
1 cup non-fat yogurt
½ cup ice cubes

Preparation: Peel and slice the banana, then place it in a blender with the apple, yogurt, and ice cubes. Blend until smooth.
Storage: Store in the refrigerator and consume within 24 hours.

7. Strawberry Almond Smoothie:

Ingredients:
½ cup strawberries
½ cup almond milk
1 teaspoon honey
½ cup ice cubes

Preparation: Wash the strawberries, then place them in a blender with the almond milk, honey, and ice cubes. Blend until smooth.

Storage: Store in the refrigerator and consume within 24 hours.

8. Peach Oat Smoothie:

Ingredients:
½ cup peach
½ cup oats
1 cup non-fat yogurt
½ cup ice cubes

Preparation: Peel and slice the peach, then place it in a blender with the oats, yogurt, and ice cubes. Blend until smooth.

Storage: Store in the refrigerator and consume within 24 hours.

9. Kiwi Avocado Smoothie:

Ingredients:

½ cup kiwi

½ avocado

1 cup non-fat yogurt

½ cup ice cubes

Preparation: Peel and slice the kiwi, then place it in a blender with the avocado, yogurt, and ice cubes. Blend until smooth.

Storage: Store in the refrigerator and consume within 24 hours.

10. Banana Spinach Smoothie:

Ingredients:

½ cup ripe banana

1 cup spinach

1 cup non-fat yogurt

½ cup ice cubes

Preparation: Peel and slice the banana, then place it in a blender with the spinach, yogurt, and ice cubes. Blend until smooth.

Storage: Store in the refrigerator and consume within 24 hours.

11. Mango Coconut Yogurt Smoothie:
Ingredients:
½ cup mango
½ cup coconut milk
1 cup non-fat yogurt
½ cup ice cubes
Preparation: Peel and slice the mango, then place it in a blender with the coconut milk, yogurt, and ice cubes. Blend until smooth.

Storage: Store in the refrigerator and consume within 24 hours.

12. Pineapple Banana Smoothie:
Ingredients:
½ cup ripe banana
½ cup pineapple

1 cup non-fat yogurt
½ cup ice cubes

Preparation: Peel and slice the banana, then place it in a blender with the pineapple, yogurt, and ice cubes. Blend until smooth.

Storage: Store in the refrigerator and consume within 24 hours.

13. Avocado Berry Smoothie:
Ingredients:
½ avocado
½ cup blueberries
½ cup raspberries
1 cup non-fat yogurt

Preparation: Peel and slice the avocado, then place it in a blender with the blueberries, raspberries, and yogurt. Blend until smooth.

Storage: Store in the refrigerator and consume within 24 hours.

14. Carrot Pineapple Smoothie:

<u>Ingredients:</u>
1 cup carrot juice
½ cup pineapple
1 cup non-fat yogurt
½ cup ice cubes

<u>Preparation:</u> Place the carrot juice, pineapple, yogurt, and ice cubes in a blender. Blend until smooth.

<u>Storage:</u> Store in the refrigerator and consume within 24 hours.

15. Grapefruit Mango Smoothie:

<u>Ingredients:</u>
½ cup grapefruit juice
½ cup mango
1 cup non-fat yogurt
½ cup ice cubes

<u>Preparation:</u> Place the grapefruit juice, mango, yogurt, and ice cubes in a blender. Blend until smooth.

<u>Storage:</u> Store in the refrigerator and consume within 24 hours.

16. Peach Blueberry Smoothie:

<u>Ingredients:</u>
½ cup ripe peach
½ cup blueberries,

1 cup non-fat yogurt
½ cup ice cubes

<u>Preparation:</u> Peel and slice the peach, then place it in a blender with the blueberries, yogurt, and ice cubes. Blend until smooth.

<u>Storage:</u> Store in the refrigerator and consume within 24 hours.

17. Apple Spinach Smoothie:

<u>Ingredients:</u>
1 cup spinach
½ cup apple
1 cup non-fat yogurt

½ cup ice cubes

Preparation: Wash and remove the stems from the spinach, then place in a blender with the apple, yogurt, and ice cubes. Blend until smooth.

Storage: Store in the refrigerator and consume within 24 hours.

18. Banana Almond Smoothie:

Ingredients:
½ cup ripe banana
½ cup almond milk
1 teaspoon honey
½ cup ice cubes

Preparation: Peel and slice the banana, then place it in a blender with the almond milk, honey, and ice cubes. Blend until smooth.

Storage: Store in the refrigerator and consume within 24 hours.

19. Kiwi Coconut Smoothie:

<u>Ingredients:</u>

½ cup kiwi

½ cup coconut milk

1 cup non-fat yogurt

½ cup ice cubes

<u>Preparation:</u> Peel and slice the kiwi, then place it in a blender with the coconut milk, yogurt, and ice cubes. Blend until smooth.

<u>Storage:</u> Store in the refrigerator and consume within 24 hours.

20. Orange Avocado Smoothie:

<u>Ingredients:</u>

½ cup orange juice

½ avocado

1 cup non-fat yogurt

½ cup ice cubes

<u>Preparation:</u> Peel and slice the avocado, then place it in a blender with the orange juice, yogurt, and ice cubes. Blend until smooth.

Storage: Store in the refrigerator and consume within 24 hours.

21. Mango Oat Smoothie:

Ingredients:
½ cup mango
½ cup oats
1 cup non-fat yogurt
½ cup ice cubes

Preparation: Peel and slice the mango, then place it in a blender with the oats, yogurt, and ice cubes. Blend until smooth.

Storage: Store in the refrigerator and consume within 24 hours.

22. Strawberry Banana Smoothie:

Ingredients:
½ cup ripe banana
½ cup strawberries
1 cup non-fat yogurt
½ cup ice cubes

Preparation: Peel and slice the banana, then place it in a blender with the strawberries, yogurt, and ice cubes. Blend until smooth.

Storage: Store in the refrigerator and consume within 24 hours.

23. Apple Coconut Yogurt Smoothie:
Ingredients:
½ cup apple
½ cup coconut milk
1 cup non-fat yogurt
½ cup ice cubes

Preparation: Peel and slice the apple, then place it in a blender with the coconut milk, yogurt, and ice cubes. Blend until smooth.

Storage: Store in the refrigerator and consume within 24 hours.

24. Grapefruit Banana Smoothie:
Ingredients:
½ cup ripe banana

½ cup grapefruit juice
1 cup non-fat yogurt
½ cup ice cubes

Preparation: Peel and slice the banana, then place it in a blender with the grapefruit juice, yogurt, and ice cubes. Blend until smooth.

Storage: Store in the refrigerator and consume within 24 hours.

25. Avocado Pineapple Smoothie:
Ingredients:
½ avocado
½ cup pineapple
1 cup non-fat yogurt
½ cup ice cubes

Preparation: Peel and slice the avocado, then place it in a blender with the pineapple, yogurt, and ice cubes. Blend until smooth.

Storage: Store in the refrigerator and consume within 24 hours.

26. Carrot Orange Smoothie:

Ingredients:
1 cup carrot juice
½ cup orange juice,
1 cup non-fat yogurt
½ cup ice cubes

Preparation: Place the carrot juice, orange juice, yogurt, and ice cubes in a blender. Blend until smooth.

Storage: Store in the refrigerator and consume within 24 hours.

27. Peach Almond Smoothie:

Ingredients:
½ cup ripe peach
½ cup almond milk
1 teaspoon honey
½ cup ice cubes

Preparation: Peel and slice the peach, then place it in a blender with the almond milk, honey, and ice cubes. Blend until smooth.

Storage: Store in the refrigerator and consume within 24 hours.

28. Raspberry Coconut Smoothie:

Ingredients:
½ cup raspberries
½ cup coconut milk
1 cup non-fat yogurt
½ cup ice cubes

Preparation: Place the raspberries, coconut milk, yogurt, and ice cubes in a blender. Blend until smooth.

Storage: Store in the refrigerator and consume within 24 hours.

29. Banana Mango Smoothie:

Ingredients:
½ cup ripe banana

½ cup mango
1 cup non-fat yogurt
½ cup ice cubes

<u>Preparation</u>: Peel and slice the banana, then place it in a blender with the mango, yogurt, and ice cubes. Blend until smooth.

<u>Storage</u>: Store in the refrigerator and consume within 24 hours.

30. Apple Kale Smoothie:
<u>Ingredients</u>:
½ cup apple
1 cup kale
1 cup non-fat yogurt
½ cup ice cubes

<u>Preparation</u>: Peel and slice the apple, then place it in a blender with the kale, yogurt, and ice cubes. Blend until smooth.

<u>Storage</u>: Store in the refrigerator and consume within 24 hours.

31. Blueberry Avocado Smoothie:

Ingredients:
½ cup blueberries
½ avocado
1 cup non-fat yogurt
½ cup ice cubes

Preparation: Peel and slice the avocado, then place it in a blender with the blueberries, yogurt, and ice cubes. Blend until smooth.

Storage: Store it in the refrigerator and consume it within 24 hours.

32. Peach Raspberry Smoothie:

Ingredients:
½ cup ripe peach
½ cup raspberries
1 cup non-fat yogurt
½ cup ice cubes

<u>Preparation:</u> Peel and slice the peach, then place it in a blender with the raspberries, yogurt, and ice cubes. Blend until smooth.

<u>Storage:</u> Store it in the refrigerator and consume it within 24 hours.

33. Orange Spinach Smoothie:
<u>Ingredients:</u>
1 cup spinach
½ cup orange juice
1 cup non-fat yogurt
½ cup ice cubes

<u>Preparation:</u> Wash and remove the stems from the spinach, then place in a blender with the orange juice, yogurt, and ice cubes. Blend until smooth.

<u>Storage:</u> Store it in the refrigerator and consume it within 24 hours.

34. Kiwi Banana Smoothie:
<u>Ingredients:</u>

½ cup ripe banana
½ cup kiwi
1 cup non-fat yogurt
½ cup ice cubes

Preparation: Peel and slice the banana, then place it in a blender with the kiwi, yogurt, and ice cubes. Blend until smooth.

Storage: Store it in the refrigerator and consume it within 24 hours.

35. Mango Almond Smoothie:

Ingredients:
½ cup mango
½ cup almond milk
1 teaspoon honey
½ cup ice cubes

Preparation: Peel and slice the mango, then place it in a blender with the almond milk, honey, and ice cubes. Blend until smooth.

Storage: Store it in the refrigerator and consume it within 24 hours.

36. Avocado Pineapple Yogurt Smoothie:

Ingredients:
½ avocado
½ cup pineapple
1 cup non-fat yogurt
½ cup ice cubes

Preparation: Peel and slice the avocado, then place it in a blender with the pineapple, yogurt, and ice cubes. Blend until smooth.

Storage: Store it in the refrigerator and consume it within 24 hours.

37. Grapefruit Coconut Smoothie:

Ingredients:
½ cup grapefruit juice
½ cup coconut milk
1 cup non-fat yogurt
½ cup ice cubes

Preparation: Place the grapefruit juice, coconut milk, yogurt, and ice cubes in a blender. Blend until smooth.

Storage: Store it in the refrigerator and consume it within 24 hours.

38. Banana Oat Smoothie:

Ingredients:
½ cup ripe banana
½ cup oats
1 cup non-fat yogurt
½ cup ice cubes

Preparation: Peel and slice the banana, then place it in a blender with the oats, yogurt, and ice cubes. Blend until smooth.

Storage: Store it in the refrigerator and consume it within 24 hours.

39. Apple Avocado Smoothie:

Ingredients:
½ cup apple

½ avocado
1 cup non-fat yogurt
½ cup ice cubes

Preparation: Peel and slice the apple, then place it in a blender with the avocado, yogurt, and ice cubes. Blend until smooth.

Storage: Store in the refrigerator and consume within 24 hours.

40. Strawberry Banana Yogurt Smoothie:

Ingredients:
½ cup ripe banana
½ cup strawberries
1 cup non-fat yogurt
½ cup ice cubes

Preparation: Peel and slice the banana, then place it in a blender with the strawberries, yogurt, and ice cubes. Blend until smooth.

Storage: Store in the refrigerator and consume within 24 hours.

41. Pineapple-Coconut Smoothie:

Ingredients:

-1 cup pineapple, fresh or frozen

-1/2 cup coconut milk

-2 tablespoons honey

-1/4 teaspoon ground ginger

Preparation: Put all the ingredients into a blender, then blend until smooth. Serve immediately.

Storage: Store in the refrigerator and consume within 24 hours.

42. Orange Coconut Smoothie:

Ingredients:

½ cup orange juice

½ cup coconut milk

1 cup non-fat yogurt

½ cup ice cubes

Preparation: Place the orange juice, coconut milk, yogurt, and ice cubes in a blender. Blend until smooth.

Storage: Store in the refrigerator and consume within 24 hours.

43. Raspberry Banana Smoothie:

Ingredients:
½ cup ripe banana
½ cup raspberries
1 cup non-fat yogurt
½ cup ice cubes

Preparation: Peel and slice the banana, then place it in a blender with the raspberries, yogurt, and ice cubes. Blend until smooth.

Storage: Store in the refrigerator and consume within 24 hours.

44. Avocado Banana Yogurt Smoothie:

Ingredients:
½ cup ripe banana

½ avocado
1 cup non-fat yogurt
½ cup ice cubes

Preparation: Peel and slice the banana, then place it in a blender with the avocado, yogurt, and ice cubes. Blend until smooth.

Storage: Store in the refrigerator and consume within 24 hours.

45. Spinach-Kale Smoothie:

Ingredients:
1 cup spinach, fresh or frozen
½cup kale, fresh or frozen
½ cup almond or oat milk
2 tablespoons honey
¼ teaspoon ground cinnamon

Preparation: Put all the ingredients into a blender, then blend until smooth. Serve immediately.

<u>Storage:</u> Store in the refrigerator and consume within 24 hours.

46. Pear-Cucumber Apple Smoothie:

<u>Ingredients:</u>
½ cup pear, fresh or frozen
½ cup cucumber, peeled and chopped
½ cup apple, peeled, cored, and chopped
½ cup almond or oat milk
2 tablespoons honey
¼ teaspoon ground nutmeg

<u>Preparation:</u> Put all the ingredients into a blender, then blend until smooth. Serve immediately.

<u>Storage:</u> Store in the refrigerator and consume within 24 hours.

47. Cinnamon Blueberry Smoothie:

<u>Ingredients:</u>
1 cup blueberries, fresh or frozen
½ cup almond or oat milk

2 tablespoons honey
¼ teaspoon ground cinnamon

Preparation: Put all the ingredients into a blender, then blend until smooth. Serve immediately.

Storage: Store in the refrigerator and consume within 24 hours.

48. Almond Orange-Ginger Smoothie:

Ingredients:
½ cup almond butter
½ cup freshly squeezed orange juice
¼ teaspoon ground ginger
2 tablespoons honey

Preparation: Put all the ingredients into a blender, then blend until smooth. Serve immediately.

Storage: Store in the refrigerator and consume within 24 hours.

49. Strawberry-Coconut Smoothie:
<u>Ingredients:</u>
1 cup strawberries, fresh or frozen
½ cup coconut milk
2 tablespoons honey
¼ teaspoon ground cardamom

<u>Preparation:</u> Put all the ingredients into a blender, then blend until smooth. Serve immediately.

<u>Storage:</u> Store in the refrigerator and consume within 24 hours.

50. Blueberry-Ginger Smoothie:
<u>Ingredients:</u>
1 cup blueberries, fresh or frozen
½ cup almond or oat milk
2 tablespoons honey
¼ teaspoon ground ginger

Preparation: Put all the ingredients into a blender, then blend until smooth. Serve immediately.

Storage: Store in the refrigerator and consume within 24 hours.

51. Coconut-Mango Smoothie:
Ingredients:
½ cup mango, fresh or frozen
½ cup coconut milk
2 tablespoons honey
¼ teaspoon ground cardamom

Preparation: Put all the ingredients into a blender, then blend until smooth. Serve immediately.

Storage: Store it in the refrigerator and consume it within 24 hours.

52. Banana-Cocoa Smoothie:
Ingredients:
½ cup banana, fresh or frozen

½ cup almond or oat milk
2 tablespoons cocoa powder
2 tablespoons honey

<u>Preparation:</u>Put all the ingredients into a blender, then blend until smooth. Serve immediately.

<u>Storage:</u> Store it in the refrigerator and consume it within 24 hours.

53. Orange-Almond Smoothie:

<u>Ingredients:</u>
½ cup freshly squeezed orange juice
½ cup almond butter
2 tablespoons honey
¼ teaspoon ground nutmeg

<u>Preparation:</u> Put all the ingredients into a blender, then blend until smooth. Serve immediately.

<u>Storage:</u> Store it in the refrigerator and consume it within 24 hours.

54. Banana-Cherry Blast Smoothie:

<u>Ingredients:</u>

½ cup banana, fresh or frozen

½ cup cherries, fresh or frozen

½ cup almond or oat milk

2 tablespoons honey

¼ teaspoon ground cinnamon

<u>Preparation:</u> Put all the ingredients into a blender, then blend until smooth. Serve immediately.

<u>Storage:</u> Store it in the refrigerator and consume it within 24 hours.

55. Apple-Mint Refresher Smoothie:

<u>Ingredients:</u>

½ cup apple, peeled, cored, and chopped

½ cup freshly squeezed orange juice

2 tablespoons honey

¼ teaspoon ground mint

<u>Preparation:</u> Put all the ingredients into a blender, then blend until smooth. Serve immediately.

<u>Storage:</u> Store it in the refrigerator and consume it within 24 hours.

56. Orange-Kale-Ginger Detox Smoothie:
<u>Ingredients:</u>
½ cup freshly squeezed orange juice
½ cup kale, fresh or frozen
¼ teaspoon ground ginger
2 tablespoons honey

<u>Preparation:</u> Put all the ingredients into a blender, then blend until smooth. Serve immediately.

<u>Storage:</u> Store it in the refrigerator and consume it within 24 hours.

57. Coconut-Blueberry Dream Smoothie:

<u>Ingredients:</u>
1 cup blueberries, fresh or frozen
½ cup coconut milk
2 tablespoons honey
¼ teaspoon ground nutmeg

<u>Preparation:</u> Put all the ingredients into a blender, then blend until smooth. Serve immediately.

<u>Storage:</u> Store it in the refrigerator and consume it within 24 hours.

58. Pineapple-Cucumber Pick-Me-Up Smoothie:

<u>Ingredients:</u>
½ cup pineapple, fresh or frozen
½ cup cucumber, peeled and chopped
¼ teaspoon ground cardamom

<u>Preparation:</u> Put all the ingredients into a blender, then blend until smooth. Serve immediately.

<u>Storage:</u> Store it in the refrigerator and consume it within 24 hours.

CHAPTER 5: Tips for Making the Perfect Gastritis-Friendly Smoothie

Making a gastritis-friendly smoothie can be a great way to get in some much-needed nutrients without causing any further irritation to your digestive tract. Here are some tips to help you make the perfect gastritis-friendly smoothie:

1. Choose the right base: When it comes to making a gastritis-friendly smoothie, it is important to choose the right base. The best base for a gastritis-friendly smoothie is low-acid fruit or vegetable juice, such as apple or carrot juice. You can also use low-fat milk or almond milk as your base.

2. Add digestive-friendly ingredients: Adding ingredients that are good for digestion can help ease the symptoms of gastritis. For example, adding ginger, turmeric, and chamomile can help reduce inflammation and soothe the stomach. You can also add probiotic-rich ingredients, such as yogurt or kefir, to help balance the bacteria in your gut.

3. Skip the sugar: Refined sugar can further irritate your stomach, so it's best to avoid adding it to your smoothie. Instead, you can use natural sweeteners such as honey or maple syrup.

4. Add a fiber source: Adding a source of fiber to your smoothie can help ease digestion and make it easier for your stomach to handle the smoothie. Good sources of fiber include chia seeds, flax seeds, oats, and fruits and vegetables.

5. Avoid acidic ingredients: Certain acidic ingredients can further irritate your stomach and cause gastritis symptoms to flare up. So it's best to avoid adding ingredients like citrus fruits, tomatoes, and vinegar to your smoothie.

6. Blend, don't juice: Blending is a great way to add more fiber to your smoothie, which can help ease digestion. Juicing can strip away the fiber, so it's best to blend your smoothie instead.

Following these tips can help you make the perfect gastritis-friendly smoothie. Making a smoothie with the right ingredients can help you get the nutrients you need without irritating your stomach.

How to create the perfect gastritis smoothie consistency.

Creating the perfect gastritis smoothie consistency is all about having the right balance of ingredients. You want to make sure that the smoothie is not too thick or too thin, as this will affect the flavor and texture. Here are some tips for getting the perfect consistency for your gastritis smoothie:

1. Start with a liquid base. This could be anything from water, juice, almond milk, or coconut milk. The type of liquid you choose will depend on the flavor and texture you're looking for.

2. Add healthy fat. This could be something like avocado, nut butter, or coconut oil. The healthy fat will help to make the smoothie creamy and give it a more satisfying texture.

3. Add your favorite fruits or vegetables. You can use fresh or frozen fruits and vegetables, depending on what you have available. Make sure to choose something low in acidity, as this can irritate the stomach.

4. Add a thickener. This could be anything from chia seeds, oats, or Greek yogurt. The thickener will help to make your smoothie more creamy and give it a thicker consistency.

5. Blend everything. Use a high-speed blender to get the perfect texture. You want the consistency to be smooth and creamy, not too thin or too thick.

6. Adjust the liquid as needed. If your smoothie is too thick, you can add more liquid until you get the desired consistency.

These are some tips for creating the perfect gastritis smoothie consistency. Make sure to adjust the ingredients and liquid to your taste and dietary needs. Enjoy!

How to choose the best type of blenders for making gastritis smoothies

Choosing the best type of blender for making gastritis smoothies can seem like an overwhelming task, but it doesn't have to be. If you're looking for a blender that will make smoothies specifically for people with gastritis, there are several factors to consider.

First, consider the power of the blender. A powerful blender is essential for blending ingredients with a silky smooth consistency. If you're looking for a blender specifically for gastritis smoothies, you'll want to make sure it is at least 600 Watts. This will ensure that the blender can handle the tough ingredients you'll be blending, such as frozen fruits, vegetables, and nuts.

Second, consider the features that the blender offers. If you want to make the most out of your gastritis smoothie, you should look for a blender that has multiple speed settings. This will allow you to control the texture of the smoothie according to your needs. Another feature to look for is a pulse setting. This will allow you to add a burst of power to the blender, which can help break down tougher ingredients.

Third, consider the size of the blender. For making gastritis smoothies, you'll want to make sure that the blender is large enough to accommodate all of your ingredients. If you plan on making larger batches of smoothies, you'll need a larger blender that can hold more ingredients.

Finally, consider the price of the blender. Blenders can range in price from very affordable to very expensive. When choosing a blender for making gastritis smoothies, you'll want to make sure that you get the best bang for your buck. Make sure to read reviews to ensure that you are getting a quality product.

Information on food safety and storage for gastritis smoothies

When it comes to food safety and storage, it is important to know how to properly store and handle food to reduce the risk of foodborne illness and other health risks. Gastritis sufferers should pay special attention to their food safety and storage practices to reduce the risk of further irritation to the stomach lining.

The first step in ensuring food safety and storage is to purchase high-quality, fresh ingredients. When selecting fruits and vegetables, be sure to check for mold, bruises, and other signs of spoilage. Fruits and vegetables should be stored in a cool, dry area away from direct sunlight. Meats, dairy, and other perishable items should be kept in the refrigerator or freezer and should be consumed within the recommended time frame.

To prevent cross-contamination, store raw meats, poultry, and seafood away from other foods. It is also important to keep cutting boards and other utensils clean and separate. When preparing food, it is important to thoroughly wash all fruits and vegetables and to cook meat to the recommended temperature.

When storing and reheating foods, be sure to use containers that are made from safe materials and labeled with the date they were made. Leftovers should be stored in the refrigerator and consumed within three days, or frozen for longer storage. Any leftover smoothies should also be stored in the refrigerator and consumed within two days.

By following these food safety and storage tips, you can reduce the risk of foodborne illness and further irritation to the stomach lining. Your health is important and taking the time to properly store and handle food can help you stay healthy.

CONCLUSION

In conclusion, Smoothies for Gastritis are an excellent way to incorporate healthy foods into your diet to reduce gastritis symptoms. They are easy to make, delicious, and full of vitamins and minerals. Not only do they help reduce gastritis symptoms, but they can also provide a much-needed energy boost throughout the day. Smoothies are also a great way to get your daily fiber intake and help keep your digestive system regular. As always, it is important to discuss any new dietary changes with your doctor or dietitian to ensure that any new foods are suitable for your condition. Smoothies can be a great addition to any gastritis diet, and with a few simple ingredients, you can make a nutritious and delicious smoothie that will help you feel better and stay healthy.

Remember, no matter what condition you have, taking steps to reduce symptoms and stay healthy is always a good choice. Smoothies for Gastritis are a great way to do just that. Enjoy!

Also, although Smoothies for Gastritis can help reduce symptoms and provide important nutrients, it's important to note that these smoothies should not replace any prescribed treatments for gastritis. Be sure to consult your doctor or dietitian about any changes to your diet and to make sure that you are still getting the nutrients you need.

Furthermore, the recipes provided in this book are just a few examples of how you can incorporate smoothies into your diet. Feel free to experiment and find your favorite smoothie recipes. There is no right or wrong way to make a smoothie, so have fun and enjoy the process.

Overall, Smoothies for Gastritis are an excellent way to get essential vitamins and minerals while also reducing symptoms of gastritis. They are easy to make, delicious, and can provide an energy boost throughout the day. By following a few simple steps and consulting your doctor or dietitian, you can add smoothies to your diet and enjoy the many benefits they provide.

So grab a blender and get started on your smoothie journey today!